The Good Cancer

The Good, The Bad, The Ugly

By Dr. Marla Friedman
Edited by Julie Tarman

Copyright

Table of Contents

Acknowledgments

Everyone has a story.

This is my story of how I was diagnosed with cancer twice. The first time in my 20s and the second time in my 40s. Everyone's cancer journey is different. This story is about coping, survival, and moving forward. This book is dedicated to my family, including my husband Marc who has supported me through six surgeries and treatment over the past 20 years. The committed healthcare professionals I have met along the way were for the most part skilled and caring. I am grateful for the oncologists, endocrinologists, radiologists, anesthesiologists, surgeons, and nurses who tirelessly deal with the big "C" each day.

This project would not have come to fruition without the encouragement of my friend and business coach Peter Marcus who asked me for three years, "Did you finish your book yet?" I would also like to acknowledge my community of friends, colleagues, students, book club, fitness trainer, yoga studio members, tennis club, and dragon boat team who continue to support me. Thank you to everyone at Story Ninjas who agreed to publish this book.

Chapter 1

Diagnosis: Shock & Awe

According to the American Cancer Society, one in three people in the U.S. will develop some type of cancer in their lifetime. When I was diagnosed with cancer the first time, I was a happy newlywed in my late 20s. It was 2001. My career in higher education was going well and I was pursuing a doctoral degree. We were enjoying our life in South Florida. My husband and I were both active and considered ourselves healthy, going to the gym every day before work and having fun in South Beach on the weekends. For no particular reason I decided to go for a physical exam, so I found a local general practitioner on the Internet. The physician was teaching his student how to conduct a thorough routine exam, which includes the doctor standing behind the patient and feeling the front of the neck area for any abnormalities. The doctor conducted the neck exam first, then the student. The physician repeated a sweep of my neck and pointed something out to the resident. I had no idea what was happening. My neck looked normal and I felt fine. Before I knew it, the doctor told me to schedule a CAT scan of my neck ASAP. I had no symptoms at all but listened to his advice. A few weeks later I was told by an endocrinologist that he had good news and bad news. The bad news: you have cancer. The good news: you have "the good cancer." The doctor assured us, "If you are going to have cancer, thyroid cancer is the one you want."

WHAT?

I didn't want *any* cancer.

Tips for Newly Diagnosed Patients

1. Don't stay up all night "Googling" your cancer. The internet can be a great tool. But it can also lead you down a slippery slope. When I couldn't sleep, I stayed up researching treatments and side effects. This is not a good idea, especially when you are first diagnosed. I found morbid stories, photos of botched surgeries, and a list of medical journal articles explaining my cancer in way too much detail. This rabbit hole is easy to fall into. Google isn't a doctor. Reading about the worse case scenario isn't helpful. Limit your time and efforts on the Internet.

2. Take a deep breath. Even though the initial diagnosis is probably shocking, remember that you are in control. Cancer medical care has progressed over the years. As a patient, you must be your own advocate. Don't be afraid to ask questions, take notes at appointments, and ask for alternative

approaches. If you are too upset to focus on what the physician is saying, bring a family member or friend to take notes for you. Come prepared with a list of questions. You can even record a physician conversation (with permission) on a phone for future reference.

3. Get a second and third opinion. If you don't feel comfortable with a physician, find another one. I have used the Internet, called support groups, and asked other patients about their experiences. When interviewing physicians, you have the right to ask them how many procedures they have performed. I asked some of my doctors if they could provide the names of former patients that I could call to speak with them about their experiences. Keep in mind that you will likely spend time in a hospital. I have had six cancer-related surgeries in five different hospitals. When choosing a physician, you are also choosing the hospital they are affiliated with. If a private room is important to you, or excellent nurses, then ask those questions. How long will you be in the hospital? All of these are valid questions. I realized through my two cancer experiences that treatment recommendations can differ greatly. For example, when I was later diagnosed with breast cancer, one oncologist suggested a lumpectomy with radiation and another was adamant that I needed a single

mastectomy, while yet another told me I needed a double mastectomy. The entire process was very confusing. How could three highly skilled physicians recommend such different protocols?

For more tips for newly diagnosed patients, check out my website (www.thegoodcancer.com)

Chapter 2

The Big "C"

My diagnosis was papillary carcinoma: the most common of the several types of thyroid cancer. Over 56,000 cases of thyroid cancer were diagnosed in the U.S. in 2017 (www.thyca.org). Papillary and follicular cancer both have a high cure rate. The standard treatment is removal of the thyroid gland. If the tumor is larger than 1 cm, then the radioactive iodine is used after surgery. Sometimes the lymph nodes need removing since the spreading of the cancer to this area is common.

I was sent for several tests to verify the CT scan by a needle biopsy (fine needle aspiration). A long needle is inserted into the neck with the hopes of extracting cells that can be tested for cancer. Not only was I awake during this procedure with just Lidocaine for the pain, I endured this test about five times. Each time the test results were "inconclusive." Imagine sticking a needle into an apple without the assurance that the needle will hit the core each time. Finally, the doctors decided that my entire thyroid had to be removed: a total thyroidectomy. The surgery was supposed to take around two hours, but after three and a half hours my family was still in the waiting room. My husband had a feeling that something wasn't right. After four hours the vascular surgeon walked into the waiting room and spoke to my husband. He said that the surgery had not gone as planned. The doctor had to scrape cancer cells off the laryngeal nerve (near the vocal cord) along with removing my entire thyroid.

My mother had a hard time accepting that her only daughter had cancer. She traveled to Florida from Connecticut and wouldn't leave my bedside in the hospital. I woke up a few times in the dark and she was sitting there. Finally the nurses asked her to leave so I could rest.

After about one week recovery time, I returned to my job as the Associate Director of International and Online Programs at a law school. I was sporting a bandage on my neck and a weak voice but I was back to my busy schedule. One day during this time my boss came into my office and sat down. He was the associate dean and the quintessential law professor with a beard and a fondness for the Renaissance. He stroked his beard and told me that he couldn't imagine how I was dealing with a cancer diagnosis. A few months later the dean was forgetting students' names and suffering from severe headaches. Six weeks after that he died of a brain tumor. Cancer can be surprising, painful, and sometimes ironic.

Once a patient's thyroid is removed, they must take thyroid replacement medication for the rest of their life. The thyroid is like a controller for your body: regulating body temperature, weight, hormones, and energy. Without thyroid replacement you can feel exhausted. Too much and you could have heart palpitations and shaky hands. The most prescribed drug for thyroid replacement is Synthroid. There are also generic versions and natural alternatives made from pigs, although many doctors are hesitant to prescribe these since they are difficult to regulate. Another drug called Cytomel is also prescribed if blood tests reveal that the T3 and T4 thyroid levels are off. Many months of adjusting the prescriptions levels are required to determine the correct amount when first taking these. Pregnancy, aging, and other factors may require additional adjustments. Typically, blood tests are drawn every few months for new patients. I will be taking Synthroid and Cytomel daily for the rest of my life.

The doctors discussed a plan with me and my husband following surgery, and we learned that the treatment for thyroid cancer hasn't changed in over 40 years. After removing a portion or the entire thyroid, the area can be treated with radioactive iodine (RAI) to kill any remaining cancer cells. This occurs when necessary, not in all thyroid cancer cases. Usually this is administered about six to eight months following surgery. Preparation for radiation includes eating a low-iodine diet for at least two weeks prior. Limiting iodine intake is so that the lack of iodine in cells becomes useful during scans. The cells are starved of iodine, allowing the cancer cells to be either detected or destroyed. The thyroid gland uses iodine obtained by food and water to produce hormones that maintain metabolism in the body. This ensures that there is no iodine in the patient so the radioactive iodine can be most effective.

What has iodine? Any table salt except non-iodized and Kosher salt. All canned products contain iodine in the lining of the metal cans. Most beans, with the exception of non-canned garbanzo beans, are not allowed. Cruciferous vegetables, such as cauliflower and broccoli, contain iodine. No dairy products are allowed as they all have iodine, including eggs. No seafood is allowed. Any foods with red dye #3, processed foods, chocolate containing milk, and commercially baked foods are not allowed. Even shampoo with red dye should be avoided. Since restaurants typically use salt to flavor their food, eating out is not an option. A diet consisting of fruit, most vegetables, plain meats, unsalted nuts, and not much else requires proper planning. I remember having cut-up apples, nuts, and carrots on hand at all times. Thankfully, the Thyroid Cancer Survivor's Association (ThyCa) provides a low-iodine diet cookbook on their website (www.thyca.org).

Radioactive iodine treatment was an isolating experience. Depending on the dose, patients given a fair amount of RAI must be isolated since the entire body is considered radioactive. The nuclear medicine doctor administers a radioactive pill that he carries to the hospital room in a James Bond-looking silver case. Once you swallow the pill, you are left alone. The nurses were scared to come near my room. This was probably because of the giant skull and crossbones on the door that read "radioactive." Food was slid under the door to me for the two days I was in the hospital. Of course, you are not supposed to eat anything with iodine in it because that would negate the effect of the uptake of radioactive iodine into the thyroid area. However, my first meal provided was salty soup with Saltine crackers, both of which have iodized salt. The hospital was clearly not equipped for this treatment.

The only redeeming aspect was the partial ocean view the Miami Beach hospital provided, and watching the winter Olympics on TV. Incidentally, this was the same hospital I was born in before moving to Connecticut when I was two years old. After two days I was released to go home with instructions to maintain three feet of distance from my husband (or any other individuals), use a different bathroom, and use disposable silverware and plates. I was also warned to stay away from pregnant women and pets. It was unnerving to walk around the house knowing I was radioactive and worrying about exposing others to radiation. My closest friend gave birth the day I was in the hospital receiving radiation. I felt really bad when my husband went to see the baby and I was alone in a different hospital.

About a month later I returned to Miami Beach for a full body scan to be sure no cancer cells were remaining. In preparation for the test, patients are required to stop taking any thyroid hormone for one to two weeks. Sometimes you can take a drug called Thyrogen, which contains a thyroid stimulating hormone (TSH) that is an injection used during this process to detect any remaining thyroid tissue after a thyroidectomy. There is a list of side effects including fatigue, headaches, and nausea.

I remember feeling exhausted. I was so tired that I sat in my car in my neighborhood supermarket parking lot wondering how I would have the energy to drive home, 10 minutes away. When the results came in we were relieved: no signs of cancer! The surgery and radiation had worked. However, this was not the end of my cancer journey. It was only the beginning.

A known side effect of this radiation is salivary gland damage. For the first few months, food tasted metallic. My salivary glands and taste buds are still not the same since the radiation. Even now, after 17 years, food often tastes extremely salty, and vinegary or acidic foods cause swelling in my glands. Dry mouth is another symptom caused by radiation. The years of dry mouth eventually led to major tooth decay. Growing up, my parents were adamant about our teeth being cared for and straightened with braces. Last year my dentist told me that every tooth in my entire mouth was suffering from enamel decay from dry mouth and needed to be replaced with either a veneer or a crown. How could this be happening? I almost fell out of the chair when he handed me the proposed cost of the treatment. Two other dentists confirmed it: my teeth were decaying. This was beyond wanting veneers to have white teeth like the reality stars. This was serious. My former dentist and friend offered to help me with a more reasonable treatment plan. The months of painful four-hour appointments and costly bills will finally end soon. It was just another reminder of how much of a toll cancer can take.

Tips for Thyroid Cancer Patients

1. Learn about your type of thyroid cancer. Speak with patients that have been through surgery and treatment. Be prepared with a list of questions for the physician.

2. Choose a specialist. Thyroid cancer is treated by endocrinologists instead of oncologists. The challenge I experienced from the over one dozen endocrinologists I have seen over the years is that many of them mostly treat patients with diabetes

and thyroid disorders, not cancer. Typically I was the youngest patient and felt as though the other patients looked at me in the waiting room wondering what I was doing there. Eventually I learned that there are a small number of endocrinologists that specialize in thyroid cancer. One of my doctors was a two-hour drive away and was worth it.

3. If you are being treated with radiation, be sure to go on the low iodine diet. Check out the recipes on www.thyca.org. This really helped me by planning meals and snacks ahead of time. Even though cooking instead of eating can be a pain, it is worth it and only short term.

Chapter 3

Speechless in South Florida

Meanwhile, the weakness in my voice wasn't improving. This is a common side effect following a thyroidectomy. I was warned that some patients wake up with a sore throat and weak voice. After several months, my voice was not getting stronger. The doctors said it would recover. I waited and waited. It didn't improve. I was referred to a speech therapist, a lovely professional at a local university. However, after several treatments it was clear that it wasn't helping. At this point, desperate to speak normally, it was time for alternative medicine. Not being able to speak on the phone or even prompt automatic phone messages was increasingly frustrating.

Over the next 12 months I sought acupuncture, voice therapy, and Chinese medicine (tea from dead crickets). The tea smelled so bad that I had to prepare it outside on the patio and could barely drink it without gagging. Nothing helped. I was a public speaking professor who couldn't speak! I asked my vascular surgeon who performed the thyroidectomy to recommend a physician in the same hospital to fix my voice. The doctor placed a camera down my throat to see why I was having trouble speaking. The results were surprising. My left vocal cord was paralyzed. During the thyroidectomy the surgeon scraped the laryngeal nerve to remove cancer cells, inadvertently paralyzing my vocal cord in the process. After showing me images of the damaged cord, the doctor discussed options. Either he could inject silicone into the vocal cord hoping it worked or perform another surgery to place a permanent implant under the paralyzed cord. Hoping for a permanent solution, I asked the doctor how many of these surgeries he had performed. His response: "40." I said, "OK, great, so you do 40 of these surgeries each year?" "No," the physician responded. "I have performed 40 laryngoplasty surgeries over the course of my career." With that I thanked him and began looking for another surgeon.

Finally in 2002 we found a specialist in New York City who performed hundreds of laryngoplasty surgeries each year. The doctor practiced at the Grabscheid Voice Center, which was created by Broadway performers in the 1940s. Patients must use their voice in their occupation in order to be eligible for treatment. Thankfully being a public speaking professor was enough to qualify. The surgeon placed a piece of silicone under my paralyzed vocal cord. During the surgery I was awake since my vocal cord had to be "tuned" by asking me to speak while it was being placed. After one night in the hospital, I stayed in NYC for 10 days for recovery. My mother-in-law asked her good friend if we could stay in her luxurious Upper East Side apartment that she wasn't using. During that time I wasn't allowed to speak at all. My mother-in-law purchased an Etch A Sketch so I could communicate. We spent time wandering around Bloomingdale's, playing Scrabble, and watching Harry Potter. She also stocked the apartment with her favorite New York City black and white treat: Mallomars. I'm pretty sure those were more for her than me. Patients are tested in a sound studio before and after surgery to record the results. Following recovery, my voice was restored to about 90% of its original strength. Today my sons are fortunate to have a mom who isn't allowed to shout.

Tips for Preventing Vocal & Salivary Gland Damage

1. Be a patient patient—your voice could recover on its own. About 5-10% of patients experience a weak or high pitch voice after thyroidectomy surgery. This can take up to six months to return to normal. If after six months the vocal changes don't improve, an ENT can diagnose the problem.

2. According to the American Thyroid Association, 10% of patients treated with high doses of radioactive iodine suffer from inflammation of the

salivary glands, dry mouth, and subsequent dental problems. Using lemon lozenges, vitamins E and C, and chewing gum may help to help protect salivary glands. https://www.thyroid.org/patient-thyroid-information/ct-for-patients/may-2018/vol-11-issue-5-p-3-4

3. Find a qualified surgeon and ask about risk of vocal damage.

Chapter 4

Cancer-Causing Exposures

According to the American Cancer Society, thyroid cancer is commonly associated with environmental causes such as exposure to radiation or various toxins. Other causes are random gene mutations and occur three times more often in women than men. (American Cancer Society - www.cancer.org.) When I was first diagnosed, my parents convinced me to see a doctor in Hartford, Connecticut, at their favorite hospital. Most of the older patients in this endocrinologist's office spoke Russian. I knew there were a fair share of Russian residents in Connecticut. What I didn't realize was that these people were survivors of the Chernobyl reactor accident in 1986. According to the UN's Scientific Committee on the Effects of Atomic Radiation report in 2011, more than 6,000 citizens living near Chernobyl (now part of Ukraine) were diagnosed with thyroid cancer. This was one of the worst nuclear disasters in human history. In fact, 400 times more radiation was spread in the air in Chernobyl than in Hiroshima when the atomic bomb was dropped during WWII. In the western United States, atomic bombs were tested in the 1950s and many of the nearby residents were exposed to harmful radiation at much lower levels than Chernobyl, and also were diagnosed with thyroid cancer. (https://www.endocrineweb.com/news/thyroid-cancer/4780-un-releases-report-chernobyl-survivors-thyroid-cancer)

So why is this relevant?

The small picturesque Connecticut town I grew up in was very far from Chernobyl. When I was diagnosed I started speaking to friends and neighbors. My high school friend had thyroid cancer as an adult, my next door neighbor growing up had thyroid cancer, and my father had thyroid nodules removed. When I learned this, I started conducting research. Another environmental cause of thyroid cancer is contaminated drinking water. Growing up we did what everyone else did—drank tap water, and a lot of it. My parents didn't allow soda or other sugary drinks in the house. The drinking water in my town came from the town well. How could a New England town in this picturesque affluent area be polluted?

The town is also the home of the oldest explosives manufacturer in the United States—originally a British company that relocated to Connecticut in 1836. They actually made explosives for the Civil War. Today they are still in business—creating hardware and energetic systems for spacecraft and the military. When I was a kid I remember hearing booming noises on occasion, like bombs were going off. Sometimes the windows on our house rattled. The residents in our town knew that this was our local company testing their goods in the "Powder Forest." Guess what happens when explosives are tested? There is a by-product produced called perchlorate that can seep into the groundwater. After a bit of research, I was able to locate old EPA reports that mentioned trace amounts of perchlorate in the town water supply. Although that is a plausible cause for my cancer, it is not rock solid evidence and I'm not Erin Brockovich.

This is not the only environmental cause to blame. Excessive high-energy radiation from X-rays can also cause thyroid cancer. I had many X-rays as a child from extensive dental work and frequent sprained ankles. I don't think I'll ever know for sure how or why I got thyroid cancer but I do know all types of cancer are on the rise.

Our homes have a certain amount of radiation from electromagnetic fields caused by WiFi, microwave ovens and other sources. What can we do? Tests for radiation are available for your home. Limit your microwave oven usage. The research varies on the health effects of microwaves from low-rate radiation emitted to carcinogens leaked into your food when microwaving plastic containers. Some studies also suggest that the nutrients from vegetables are

zapped out during the microwave process.
https://www.cancer.org/cancer/cancer-causes/radiation-exposure/extremely-low-frequency-radiation.htm

I can only wonder if environmental factors could be to blame? I recently heard an interview with a physician/cancer patient advocate who said that there is a chemical coating on paper receipts that we are handed from any retail store. This coating contains a carcinogen. He suggested washing our hands if we have to touch these receipts. Wow. As I drove down the road listening to this interview I couldn't help but think about the thousands of receipts I have handled over the years. Another news story just released states that Cheerios and other oat based products contain trace amounts of weed killer, which is a carcinogen. Other reports cite that the plastic from our bottled water contains BPA, causes rises in estrogen levels in women and may lead to cancer.
https://www.breastcancer.org/risk/factors/plastic Is this why I had cancer?

Many of us have heard about other environmental factors that may lead to cancer such as plastics and red dye. In fact, red dye #3 was already banned by the FDA in 1990 for use in cosmetic and topical drugs since it can cause thyroid tumors. (www.thetruthaboutcancer.com) However, the carcinogen continues to be widely used in foods such as Maraschino cherries, popsicles, and sausage. The FDA ban on food additives for red dye #3 has been postponed over 26 times due to pressure from the food industry. Thinking about all of our cancer risks can be overwhelming. Throughout college I sold cellular phones when they first hit the market, beginning with the famous "brick phone." Since cell phones emit radioactive waves, there has been talk for years about the risk of cell phone use. When I sold phones at a kiosk in Boston, people used to come to my booth just to tell me that my ear was going to fall off from using these new mobile devices. Thankfully that hasn't happened and the research about cell phone use isn't clear. I am careful about having my phone next to my head too much and try to use headphones or Bluetooth. A recent study of 9-11 first responders reported many being diagnosed with thyroid cancer. At some point it can create even more stress in our lives by worrying about what could be. However, making the best choices we can for ourselves and our families based on the information we have available is the best we can do.

Tips for Improving Your Environment

1. Avoid excessive X-rays. Always ask for a thyroid shield during imaging. Even though X-ray technology has improved, you can never be too careful.

2. Create a healthy home by limiting mold exposure, dust, and chemicals. We have two medical grade air purifiers in our home. This cleans air pollutants and filters viruses and bacteria. We also have a humidifier which helps with allergies and sinus issues. Using organic cleaning products is helpful since most products contain many toxic chemicals.

3. Be sure drinking water is tested and safe, or use bottled water. Also, installing a reverse osmosis filter in your home is a viable solution, as is using refillable bottles. Both will save money in the long run.

Chapter 5

Socrates Café

At any age, a cancer diagnosis can make you question your own mortality. At 29 years old I was asking a lot of questions.

Why me?

Why now?

What did I do to get cancer?

Why are some people at an early age given an early exit?

I started reading books on philosophy. *The Socrates Café* by Christopher Phillips was an easy read about a group of people across the U.S. who read the teachings of Socrates and met at libraries to discuss the principles. I loved this concept and was always enthralled with philosophical questions starting with my introduction to existentialism in my high school English class when we read *Waiting for Godot.*

Another weighty topic I was drawn to was the Holocaust. I read *The Diary of Anne Frank* when I was younger. I began reading *Night* by Elie Wiesel and other stories of people suffering. I'm not sure what my attraction to this genre was at the time. Perhaps I wanted to know that all people go through hardships. My late grandmother Goldie Gold (her real name) had a saying: if you took your problems and put them in a basket, and someone else's problems and placed them in a different basket, you would always choose your own basket.

I re-read *You Can Heal Your Life* by Louise Hay. Although written in the 1980s, some of the wisdom still holds true: we can manifest feelings and experiences. Negative thoughts can actually turn into disease such as cancer. Other books I was drawn to include *The Secret* and *The Celestine Prophecy*. It's all about manifesting your own destiny. According to self-help author Wayne Dyer, we don't have to believe every thought we have. We have the power to manage our thoughts, feelings, and emotions. The law of attraction can also work for our overall health.

Tips for Handling Cancer

1. Read stories of inspiration, personal achievement, or even trashy novels if that makes you happy.

2. Listen to music. Music can have a positive influence on emotions. Relaxing music while waiting to see a doctor or uplifting music on a bad day can always help. I listened to a special meditation for surgery that I purchased and placed on an iPod for each procedure. The doctors had no

problem wheeling me into the operating room wearing headphones.

3. Laugh—watch a comedy. Humor can help you get through tough times. Watching a stand-up special on TV, or going to a comedy club or watching a funny film can improve your mood. This plan backfired a little when I was watching a stand-up comedienne on TV thinking I would escape thinking about cancer for an hour. All of a sudden she began talking about being diagnosed with breast cancer, then proceeded to take her shirt off showing her mastectomy scars to the audience. It was refreshing and slightly shocking how this comic was so honest and making jokes about her own experience. Laughter can be the best medicine.

Chapter 6

I'm Still Here—A Survivor

Following radioactive iodine, women are instructed to wait for at least 12 months before becoming pregnant to be sure that the toxins are out of the body. I had already been married for four years. Although we weren't ready to start a family before cancer, when you are told you aren't allowed to do something, somehow you suddenly want it. It seemed like everyone around me was having babies. All of our friends and neighbors were either pregnant, breast feeding, or potty training their toddlers. I felt as though these women were in a club in which I wasn't a member, even if it was short term. Once the one-year mark after radiation passed, my husband and I decided to begin trying for a family and I became pregnant right away. We were excited and relieved! I was 30 years old, we were building a house, and my career was going well. Since I am the older sibling, this would be my parent's first grandchild. Before even becoming pregnant I had signed up to take a motorcycle license course and compete on a tennis league. I accomplished both while pregnant.

Thankfully I loved being pregnant and did not suffer from any side effects.

Once I recovered from thyroid cancer in 2002, I wanted to prove to myself that cancer wouldn't stop me. I signed up for a 150-mile bike ride from Miami to Key Largo even though I had never cycled for more than 30 miles. Before I could think about competing I needed to train so I joined a local riding group. The first day riding with a group I showed up with my Cannondale mountain bike. In the first 30 minutes, the entire group was miles ahead of me on their sleek and lightweight road bikes and I felt embarrassed and exhausted wondering what I was doing. The spinning classes at my gym had not prepared me for the road. This was different. I purchased a road bike, compiled a team from my university, trained each Sunday by riding 60 miles with a group, raised money for the MS Association, and felt accomplished.

The day of the ride my friend picked me up at four a.m. to drive one hour to Miami with our bikes. At the start my friend took off with some other team members at a fast pace. I was sticking together with another rider since our pace was similar. In the back of my mind I was worried about falling and possible hurting my unborn child during the 150-mile ride. Somehow I figured this wouldn't stop me. About two hours into the ride, I looked up and saw something that wasn't rain falling out of the sky. It was hail! All of a sudden, hail started pounding us. Ride organizers were driving around in trucks picking up riders who had enough. My riding partner asked if I wanted to stop. My response: absolutely not! I just beat cancer, trained for six months, and wasn't going to let a little hail stop me from finishing. Hours later I was wet, bruised from the hail, and tired. Struggling up over the gradual incline of the Card Sound Road bridge in Key Largo was a challenge. Floridians aren't used to hills! The feeling of accomplishment coasting down the other side nearing the finish line was immeasurable.

One week after completing the ride, I flew to New York City for another bike ride with my father and brother called Bike New York. At a family dinner before the event, I handed my parents a photo frame of my ultrasound as a surprise, announcing to my parents that we were expecting our first child (their first grandchild). Everyone was so excited!

The next morning me, my father, and brother biked through the streets of Manhattan, planning to travel over 50 miles through all five boroughs. The ride began at the World Trade Center, headed uptown, then entered Central Park. There were thousands of riders converging into the park at the same time, sometimes making maneuvering a challenge. My brother had to swerve his wheel into mine for a split second avoiding another biker, causing us both to crash. My brother's hand was bleeding and although I felt fine we were both taken by ambulance to the nearest hospital with my father. The Bike New York personnel told us they would lock up our bikes which we could retrieve later. Since I was five weeks pregnant, the hospital suggested an examination. After four hours in the emergency room with gunshot victims and a criminal who was handcuffed to a stretcher, my brother was released with a sprained arm and given a sling. My musician brother wouldn't be able to play his guitar for a while. I was checked and had no injuries. At this point my father wanted to eat so we proceeded to the Carnegie Deli where he enjoyed corned beef on rye. After showing up at the designated area in Central Park for the three bikes, it was clear that they were not there. The NYPD filed a theft report. We spent the next several hours in our Spandex and cycling shoes, searching in different Bike New York facilities around the city. The bikes were never to be found and likely had been stolen.

Driving to the airport to go home with my mother the next day, I began having severe cramps. Since my mother had been through several miscarriages and difficult pregnancies I asked if this was normal. Silence followed. She looked at me in a way that indicated "this isn't a good sign." We said goodbye as she apprehensively dropped me off. I called my doctor from the airport before boarding the plane to let him know that I wasn't feeling well. On the flight back to Florida, the painful cramping became unbearable and I knew something was really wrong. Sitting alone, the pain was so intense that tears were streaming down my face. The flight attendants were thoughtful and tried to help. Upon landing, my husband met me with a wheelchair and I was rushed to the ER. My OBGYN performed an emergency procedure (D&C) that surgically removes the tissue from the uterus after a miscarriage. It was extremely painful, both physically and emotionally. I had lost the baby. It was so disappointing. I'm grateful that two healthy pregnancies followed starting a year later. My sons are now teenagers and (to my disbelief) taller than me. Last year (in 2017) we participated in Bike New York as a family once again. There were no crashes this time, just fun memories. We fondly call the event "Crash New York." Bike New York taught me to seize the day, move on, and not live in fear.

Tips for Moving On

1. Find a cause. Use your own experience to help others.

2. Join/start a support group. When I was diagnosed and seeking support, I attended a group meeting in a club that operates out of South Florida. Even though everyone was welcoming, all of the women had breast cancer. I couldn't relate to their issues

and wondered why there wasn't a group for thyroid cancer patients. I looked, but couldn't find one. So, I established the first chapter of Thyca-Thyroid Cancer Survivors' Association in South Florida in 2001. My public relations background came in handy while promoting the new group which is still going strong. I continue to support newly diagnosed patients on a regular basis.

3. Try a new hobby. Keeping your mind occupied while learning something new can be fun and therapeutic. If you need some ideas, check your local Meetup.com site. Groups for everything from people with dogs who play frisbee to chess to canoeing clubs are listed. For more tips on moving on, check out my website (www.thegoodcancer.com).

Chapter 7

The Not-So-Sexy Cancer

Around my birthday I booked a mammogram as most women of a certain age do. In September of 2014 I went to my appointment and had imaging done along with an ultrasound. After having thyroid cancer, my doctor wanted me to have a diagnostic ultrasound and a mammogram. When that test was over I was happy to leave. A week later I received a letter from the hospital stating they wanted to perform a biopsy on a "suspicious" area. I went back to the hospital where they proceeded to smoosh my breast in a mammogram machine and then stick a giant needle in to withdraw a cell sample. I was apprehensive about the needle, because I had implants, and a needle near a saline-filled container is never a good idea! After the procedure I was still in the room when the radiologist showed me the sample they removed on a screen. He pointed out that the cell formation didn't appear to be cancer. I was relieved and again happy to go home. A few days later I received a phone call from a different radiologist. I was at the market buying groceries and answered the call. Since I had never even met this doctor I wondered why she was calling me.

The conversation went something like this:

"Hello. This is Doctor So-and-So. I reviewed your biopsy results. You have breast cancer."

What!?!?

She had a foreign accent and I thought maybe I heard wrong.

EXCUSE ME?

I told her that the performing radiologist told me that it didn't look like cancer. She said that the results indicated DCIS (ductal carcinoma in situ) and told me I needed another biopsy. After hanging up I stood in the parking lot next to a collection of shopping carts in complete shock.

How could this be happening?

Again...

If thyroid cancer is the good cancer, then breast cancer should be called the "not so sexy" cancer, or maybe the trendy cancer. Since one in eight women in the U.S. will be diagnosed with breast cancer; charities, fundraisers, and awareness amidst a sea of pink abounds. Thyroid cancer doesn't have the same status. Your thyroid isn't sporting a bikini or lacy bra. Your breasts are sexy. When your breasts are removed or cut—not so sexy. I was always well endowed and criticized women who wanted breast surgery. After having two children, I decided to have them lifted. The plastic surgeon told me he couldn't perform the lift without using implants. Although I told the doctor I didn't want to look like a porn star in preschool, I ended up with size D implants.

After the second biopsy I was told I needed to meet with a surgeon. On September 11, I met a referred surgeon at the same hospital. He told me that I should have a double mastectomy. My husband and I were taken off guard. A double mastectomy for non-invasive cancer that was only on one side? Why? The surgeon responded, "Well, your (nine-year-old) implants could use an upgrade anyway." Okay, asshole, I have cancer and haven't had any issues with my implants, thank you very much. With that I began looking for another surgeon. At yoga I met a woman who also had DCIS. When she heard I was newly diagnosed, she offered to take me to lunch and told me about her surgeon—a women who was Harvard-trained and recently moved to Florida from Boston. I quickly made an appointment. I liked how thorough she was and she explained everything. She recommended genetic testing for the BRCA gene. Women who test positive for this gene have a higher likelihood of being diagnosed with breast and ovarian cancer. The gene is common in women of Eastern European Jewish ancestry. Although my family has this ancestry, the genetic tests were negative. This was a surprise since both my grandmothers had breast cancer in their 60s, which was successfully surgically removed. The oncology surgeon explained that the hospital had a new machine that provided patients with radiation during surgery. Another option was that I could have a lumpectomy followed by radiation every day for six weeks. I already had radiation for thyroid cancer (which can be caused by radiation) and didn't like the sound of six weeks of radiation. Plus, the radiation can harden the implants and then encapsulate them to further complicate the situation.

I booked the surgery anyway and figured I could always opt out of the radiation. In the meantime, I continued to ask friends and family about doctors and hospitals. I met with a veteran oncologist at the University of Miami. He recommended the surgeon from Boston who I already scheduled surgery with. A friend's cousin is a radiologist at Sloan Kettering and I was given the name of a breast cancer surgeon. Since I already had one good experience with surgery in New York City and a bad experience with surgery in Florida, I decided to call Sloan Kettering. After booking an appointment for a consultation, I canceled my October surgery in Florida. Following many sleepless nights, my instincts told me that the hospital I booked in Florida just wasn't the right choice.

In the meantime, I was scheduled to speak at the Thyroid Cancer Survivor's Association International Conference in Denver, Colorado in October. My husband and I traveled to Denver for a few days and attended the conference. My speech, entitled "Ten Tips for Conquering Cancer," went over very well. I met an endocrinologist from Sloan Kettering. I asked him if there was any link between thyroid cancer and breast cancer. He said there was a possibility that the radiation from thyroid cancer treatment may have caused breast cancer.

Wow.

One thing I recommend is not to be diagnosed with breast cancer during breast cancer awareness month in October. Every hotel, hospital, and television commercial was about breast cancer. There was pink everywhere. Even Delta Airlines had pink ribbons on their napkins! We checked into the hotel in Denver and there were pink ribbons all over the lobby. What a terrific reminder that you have breast cancer!

One week later I was at Sloan Kettering in New York City. The Evelyn Lauder Breast Cancer Center is an 11-story building on the Upper East Side. My brother lives in Manhattan and met me for the appointment. The surgeon happened to be the chief of surgery for the entire center. She walked in with another female doctor (who looked like a fashion model). First, they examined me. Next, she asked me if I was seeing multiple doctors until I heard an answer that I liked. Before I could respond, she told me that I had cancer and needed surgery.

What she did next, I will never forget.

The surgeon removed a cloth tape measure from her lab coat and extended it to the four-inch mark.

"Do you see this? This is four inches. To not remove four inches of cancer would be ludicrous."

Wow.

I actually appreciated her directness. Her words convinced me to accept the diagnosis. It was exactly what I needed at that moment to make a decision about the surgery. She recommended a single mastectomy and I agreed. In the elevator my brother turned to me and said that he has never heard a physician use the word "ludicrous." He urged me to book surgery as soon as possible.

After the appointment, I went to a busy restaurant with my brother and nephew. As I was at lunch, the gravity of the news started to sink in. By the time I got to my plane, I was throwing up. I don't know if it was the mussels I ate, or the reality that this cancer was serious but the queasiness lasted for the entire two and a half hour flight back home. Good times...

I booked the surgery for December 30th when my children were on winter break and it would be easier to travel. Before the surgery I returned to New York City for a pre-op appointment and met the plastic surgeon. He was a very affable doctor and explained that he didn't recommend a single mastectomy for cosmetic reasons. I agreed that, already having implants, it made sense to remove both breasts. This also would provide peace of mind not having to worry about cancer on the right side. I went back to the cancer surgeon directly from the plastic surgeon's office. This time my mother was with me. I told the surgeon that I wanted a bilateral (double) mastectomy instead of a single. She was not happy with me since the surgery was already booked and this was around Christmas. However, they were able to change my surgery and I had a double mastectomy.

I have been to many hospitals and the care at Sloan Kettering was truly amazing. My husband and I arrived for surgery and we only waited for about five minutes before they took us into the pre-op area. A meditation for surgery audio recording was recommended to me so I listened to that on an iPod and also brought positive affirmations for the anesthesiologist to read to me. I remember being wheeled into the operating room and the doctor reading the paper and then I fell asleep. My surgery was scheduled for 11 a.m. I woke up in a plush private room and asked the nurse the time. He told me it was 9:30 p.m. How could that be? I looked around and realized that this was the nicest hospital room I had ever seen. A carpeted room with upholstered furniture, wood armoire with a flat screen TV, sleeper sofa, draperies and a view of Manhattan from the 19th floor. My male nurse was amazing. He spoke seven languages and was empathetic and warm. During the night he wanted me to go for a walk so we strolled the hallways. He pointed out the wood-paneled library with guest computers at the end of the hall. Then he showed me where visitors could take cappuccino and croissants.

"Do you see that bench in front of that door? That's for the bodyguards."

"What?"

"For when the prince stays here."

Was that the Percocet, or did he just say, "prince?" I wasn't sure which prince. The floor had two- and three-bedroom suites for patients and their entourage to stay in. This is when I realized that this was not an ordinary hospital. I was on the VIP floor of Memorial Sloan Kettering!

The next day my surgeon came to check on me wearing the most beautiful floor-length mink coat I had ever seen. Even the nurse commented that it was risky to wear mink in a hospital, but it was New Year's Eve in Manhattan. The surgeon told me that the surgery was successful and the cancer had actually spread to beyond the ducts which meant it went from non-invasive to invasive (stage 0 to stage 1.) This news convinced me that the decision of having the mastectomy versus a lumpectomy was the right choice. During the mastectomy a plastic surgeon placed tissue expanders into the breast tissue, which stayed there for 6-12 months before permanent implants were provided. Sometimes implants are placed during a mastectomy. Ask your surgeon what they recommend.

I spent the next two weeks recovering in a cousin's empty apartment. My friends in Florida called me on FaceTime from a party to wish me a healthy year. Relatives stepped in to take care of me and my children. My plans were to work on my projects, including completing this book. That didn't happen. I spent most days resting, doing my exercises, and going for walks. Most bilateral mastectomy patients will go home with drains for fluid on both sides. Patients that had a lymph node removed during the mastectomy could have from 4-6 drains following surgery. These drains speed healing include tubes from the surgical site attached to small plastic containers that must be emptied each day. If the sight of blood bothers you, be sure to designate someone to help you with this task. The drains are typically removed during your first post-surgical visit one to two weeks after surgery. The drains aren't painful but they can be uncomfortable for sleeping. Wearing loose clothing is helpful for covering the drains. Despite being in a cold climate instead of balmy South Florida in the middle of the winter, New York City is a good place to recover from surgery. Anything can be delivered and healthy food is easy to find. However, getting my arms into my winter coat proved to be challenging. My sister in law from Florida came to take care of me when my husband had to return to work. Despite the chilly temperatures and the small third-floor walk-up apartment, I have fond memories of that time spent recovering: watching the snow falling outside the window, daily walks with my sister-in-law around the Lower East Side, enjoying fresh guacamole from Whole Foods, and my brother bringing me bone broth from across town.

One day over tea my sister-in-law asked me if I had heard of an organization called Sharsheret and suggested contacting them. I followed her advice and was quickly paired with a volunteer. They also sent me an amazing array of packages including reference materials, a handmade pillow, and even a "Busy Box" with Legos and other toys for my boys—all for free! I'm truly impressed with Sharsheret. They serve a much-needed purpose serving young Jewish women with breast and ovarian cancer. I feel fortunate to have been introduced to such a well-run and supportive organization. Since then I volunteered to write a blog article about healthy living and also participated in a webinar as a patient advocate.

When it was time to return home to Palm Beach, I didn't think much about the trip. After an easy car ride to Newark, my sister-in-law and I boarded the plane. I watched the New York City skyline fade away in the dusk sky. When the plane began climbing altitude the pressure in my chest began. As we headed into the clouds the combination of the pain in my chest from the tissue expanders (probably from the cabin pressure) and the emotional pain of a double mastectomy hit me. The small airline cocktail napkins weren't large enough to wipe away the tears.

When I returned home I was followed up by a local oncologist and plastic surgeon. The tissue expanders require getting "filled" with saline for a few weeks to expand the skin. This process was extremely painful and only Lidocaine is given for the pain.

The first time I had my blood drawn by my local oncologist the nurse asked me which arm to draw from. Confused, I asked her to clarify. She told me that if I had a lymph node removed (which I did for a biopsy during the mastectomy) then I can never have blood drawn or blood pressure taken from that side ever again. This can cause inflammation and lymphedema; a blockage in the lymphatic system. Perhaps this was mentioned after the mastectomy but I had no recollection. Now when I go to a doctor or for surgery the team has to be told to only use my good arm for testing and IVs.

Even though the Sloan Kettering physician requested I take a drug called Tamoxifen, I was hesitant. The drug blocks estrogen from the body. Since my cancer was estrogen positive, it was important to keep estrogen levels low. Tamoxifen has major side effects including... cancer! There are cases (about one percent) when taking Tamoxifen causes endometrial cancer. The minor side effects of Tamoxifen are quite extensive and include early menopause, nausea, depression, mood swings, headaches, etc. The other issue with the drug is that it must be taken for five years to be effective. I wasn't ready for these side effects and the possibility of a third cancer. After calculating my low recurrence rate statistics, my local oncologist agreed to test my cancer markers every three months without taking Tamoxifen. However, during one visit to her office, a physician's assistant recommended that I go on the drug.

"Do it for your children," she said.

Really? Was she suggesting that I would die and leave my children motherless if I didn't take Tamoxifen? I explained that risking a third cancer diagnosis and suffering from debilitating side effects wasn't an option. She suggested that I reconsider, then left the room.

After that, I requested to only see my oncologist. And I stand by my decision. I always have and always will care for my health through any means possible: exercise, nutrition, stress reduction, etc. However, we all have choices to make when being treated for cancer. The process can be confusing and overwhelming. But in the end, you're the only one who has to live with the consequences.

Do your research and follow your instincts.

Tips for Mastectomy Patients

1. Ask about nipple sparing techniques. If the nipple must be removed, then inquire about skin or tattoo nipple replacement options. Some insurance companies pay for nipple tattoos and they are created using a 3D technique with amazing results. If you look online, many tattoo artists have created intricate designs on breast cancer patients. Keep in mind that after a mastectomy nerve endings are cut. You will lose most or all of the feeling in your breast and/or nipple.

2. Pack comfortable button-down shirts to wear for a week or two. Your arm movement will be limited. Be sure to do the exercises your physician recommends. This helps to avoid swelling which can cause lymphedema. This is a painful condition and can be helped by wearing a compression sleeve. Even though "wall crawls" and the other exercises I was given were the last thing I wanted to do when recuperating from surgery, I did them anyway in hopes that I could go back to playing tennis.

3. Create a healing environment for recovery. Be sure that your bedroom isn't cluttered. Use essential oils like lavender for relaxation. If you have a pet that sleeps with you like I do, make sure they don't

jump on you. This can cause serious pain and damage after surgery.

Chapter 8

What I Learned from Reconstructive Surgery

Reconstructive surgery is optional for breast cancer patients. However, according to a 2016 New York Times article, more than 106,000 reconstructive procedures were performed in 2015, a 35 percent increase since 2000.
https://www.nytimes.com/2016/11/01/well/live/going-flat-after-breast-cancer.html

Sixty-five percent of mastectomy patients between 2009 and 2014 chose reconstruction, according to the U.S. Agency for Healthcare Research and Quality (AHRQ).
https://consumer.healthday.com/cancer-information-5/breast-cancer-news-94/more-women-choose-breast-reconstruction-after-mastectomy-727397.html

Self-image can be a challenge after losing one or both breasts. Plastic surgery is more prevalent than ever. Facing reconstructive surgery following breast cancer is not the same as choosing to have implants. Removing tissue expanders and replacing them with implants for breast cancer patients can create complications. This surgery was not as painful as the mastectomy but more painful than my original implant surgery. The other factor to keep in mind is that with the breast tissue removed, the look of implants post-mastectomy can look very different. The absence of tissue can create a challenge. In total, I have had four breast surgeries. One of my friends (another survivor) likened her scars to Frankenstein. As survivors, we must accept the reality of how we look both in and out of clothes. A few times my sons have noticed my many scars and asked me about them. In their words, the scars looked "scary." I reminded them about the cancer surgery I had and told them that they don't hurt, just look ugly. That was enough of an explanation for them.

Since I was a teenager, I had large breasts. This self-identity wasn't really obvious to me for many years. When I opted for a lift after having children in my 30s, they were even larger. For 10 more years my identity of having a large chest continued. Then suddenly, after breast cancer, that was taken away. Sure, I could have asked for large implants. But felt like it wasn't' really what I wanted at this stage in my life. Sometimes, looking a photos of myself pre-breast cancer, I mourn the loss of my endowed chest. I miss having nipples and nerve endings that allow feeling. Now I can barely notice an object or a hand touching my breast since all of the nerve endings were cut in the mastectomy. Many breast cancer patients I speak with have similar sentiments. On the bright side, we are still here.

After the process of having the tissue expanders filled every week for a month by a local plastic surgeon, it was time to think about more surgery. The expanders are only meant to last from 6-12 months, and then they are traded for permanent implants. I asked for referrals so I didn't have to travel back to New York for surgery. Since plastic surgery is prevalent in South Florida, it wasn't difficult to find. However, I was seeking a plastic surgery who was proficient in reconstruction. I booked the surgery in May when my boys' school year was finishing up. The surgery went as planned and I was sent home as an outpatient the same day. As I began to heal, the results were not pleasing. I didn't like the shape and my chest was often in pain. After a year I decided I would re-do the surgery.

I yet again found another surgeon who explained what was wrong with the current implants and how he would fix them. Exactly a year after the first reconstructive surgery, I endured surgery yet again. My mother-in-law was having cancer treatment the same day, in the same hospital, coincidentally, and came to visit. The hospital experience was frustrating, with nurses who forgot to turn on my leg compression machine and never brought a wheelchair when I was discharged. My mom took a wheelchair out of the hallway herself and wheeled me to the elevator where we both declared, "Let's get out of here." Today I still am not happy with the look of the reconstructive surgery. However, I think my body needs a break from surgery for a while. The nipple tattoos will have to wait since they are permanent. If implants are replaced, the position of the tattoos won't match. After speaking with countless breast cancer patients, this is normal. Body image can really suffer after breast cancer. Although it isn't very obvious in clothes, we should be pleased with our own bodies. Lowering expectations of looking the same as before breast cancer is helpful. My husband and sons don't see me any differently and my neck scars are certainly more obvious.

For over 15 years I tried to correct the appearance of my thyroidectomy scar. It was raised, red, and sometimes painful. My olive skin is prone to keloids which is a raised and red scar caused by extra collagen in the skin. Strangers would look at my neck then stop me to ask if I had a tracheotomy. In the sun I always covered my scar and sometimes felt like a labrador retriever with a bandana around my neck. After trying steroid injections, microdermabrasion, and many creams, surgery seemed like the only solution. Over the years I asked about ten different surgeons if they could fix my scar but none of the doctors were confident they could achieve a better outcome. My endocrinologist performed an ultrasound and thankfully did not notice signs of a cancer recurrence. However, the scar had calcified underneath the skin. This caused increasing pain and redness so I began calling plastic surgeons in New York City. One surgeon asked me to text photos to decide if they would arrange a consultation. After reviewing the photos, the office responded that unfortunately they couldn't help me. However, they recommended a surgeon at NYU. After flying to New York City during spring break for a consultation, the plastic surgeon said he could successfully fix the scar. The operation went smoothly and I am looking forward to the results when it heals in a few months.

Tips for Reconstructive Surgery

1. Be realistic with your expectations. You won't look the same. Sometimes surgery can improve how you look but often you are just fixing what can be fixed.

2. Stop watching TV. Refrain from watching reality television shows like "Botched." This could cause undue anxiety and is more upsetting than helpful. There is no reason to watch plastic surgery gone wrong for entertainment.

3. Ask your surgeon what the recovery time is. Since plastic surgery is so prevalent, there is a sense that it is like having your hair done. Those of us who have gone through multiple surgeries know that surgery has side effects, pain, and a specific recovery time.

Chapter 9

What I Learned from a Dragon

Dragons are fearless.
Dragons breathe fire.
Dragons aren't afraid of cancer.

About 20 years ago, my husband and I were having dinner with his Canadian business associate and his wife. She mentioned that she was a breast cancer patient and enjoyed dragon boating. I had never heard of the sport and found the conversation interesting. She explained that the paddling motion in dragon boating was recognized to be beneficial to breast cancer survivors by a Canadian sports medicine physician. In 1996 Dr. Don McKenzie conducted research to see if upper body exercise could help prevent breast cancer patients contracting a painful condition called lymphedema. In the past, patients were advised not to do any upper body exercise. However, the women in the study became more fit and happier as a result of paddling. The camaraderie was contagious and the sport spread around the world for breast cancer survivors everywhere.

When I completed my breast cancer treatment four years ago and was ready for a new challenge, that conversation came to mind. I called the International Breast Cancer Paddle Commission (IBCPC) and asked if there was a team in Palm Beach County. Even though we are surrounded by water, there wasn't a team. I was disappointed until the person on the phone mentioned that a team member from the Miami team had moved to Palm Beach that week and was starting a new team! With no experience, I learned how to paddle and was "bit" by the dragon. After paddling only three times, I participated in my first race in Miami and was hooked. Now our team, Lighthouse Dragons SOS, has over 65 members and owns two boats. We practice twice per week in the clear blue waters of the intracoastal under the watchful eye of the historic Jupiter Lighthouse. I just returned from Florence, Italy, where our team competed in the 2018 IBCPC Dragon Boat Festival. The festival is held every four years in cities around the world during the summer. There were over 125 teams from 19 countries and every continent. Our team from Jupiter combined with a team in Melbourne, Florida to create a composite team. For several months the 26 participants practiced together to prepare.

My husband, sons, and even my business coach traveled to Italy to watch the races. After a day of practice, my team participated in a parade of nations through the streets of Florence and over the famous Ponte Vecchio bridge ending at a historic plaza for the opening ceremonies. Spectators from all over the world lined the streets cheering us on. Even the shopkeepers seemed to enjoy the festivities. Teams were grouped by country and most had a theme. Of course our Florida team was wearing red, white, and blue, flamingos, and suns. Just because we all survived cancer doesn't mean we can't have fun. Some of the international breast cancer dragon boat team names included: Prior Chestnuts, Knot a Breast, Chemo Savvy, Mamo Glams, and Missing Mammaries. Needless to say, my husband and sons were hysterically laughing while reading the names in the event program.

The race took place on a Saturday and Sunday. Our team won both heats (five boats competing) on our first day. Getting to the venue from our rented flat was an experience. Uber doesn't exist in Florence. The apartment manager tried calling me a cab. After being on hold for 20 minutes, they responded that there were no taxis available. Since time was running out I headed outside and tried to hail a taxi New York-style (even though I was told this isn't done in Florence). On the previous practice day, this had worked. This particular day, however, no taxis stopped. I headed to the bus stop and took a bus that I thought was heading in the right direction until I had to transfer buses and the new bus had broken down.

With the temperature soaring to 85 degrees Fahrenheit, I began to sweat. I started walking in the general direction of the venue. My cell phone didn't have international service so I couldn't call anyone. Wearing my team uniform of a hot pink team tank top, pink hat, lanyard with my photo, and American flag and black tights, I didn't stand out among the well-dressed Italians at all. I stopped at a hair salon asking them to call me a taxi. No taxis. I offered to pay the salon worker to drive me. She didn't have a car. I kept walking and found another bus stop. I asked someone if this was the bus to the park. He told me that it wasn't and he offered to call a taxi. However, one minute later his bus arrived. He told me to wait there since he was on the phone on hold with the taxi company and stepped onto the bus. At this point I began to panic. I just traveled thousands of miles to compete in a race. My family and friend were there to watch. My team was counting on me and time was running out. How could I be so irresponsible? I've lived in Europe and should have planned better.

Reminded by my determination to defeat cancer, I resolved to get to the race no matter what. Instead of breaking down into tears with the fear that I let my team down, I decided to remain calm. All of a sudden I saw a handsome Italian getting onto his parked Vespa. I asked him in my broken Italian if he knew which way the park was. He looked at me, handed me an extra helmet he happened to have and said in English, "Get on. I will take you." He knew about the dragon boat race. When I explained that I was quite late he told me not to worry, he could go fast through traffic. Bellissimo. He dropped me to the entrance of the park safely.

I said "grazi" and "ciao" and then realized I still had a two-mile walk to meet my team for race lineup. An American couple on bicycles saw me break into a run and offered one of their bikes. The wife told me she was also a survivor. I jumped on and she escorted me to the venue entrance where my team was waiting for me. When we won both of our races that day, it was all worth it.

Later that day, relaxing in our team tent alone, a woman asked if I would like to trade pins. Each team brings their custom designed pins to trade at every dragon boat festival. She liked our lighthouse. I asked where she was from and it turned out she was on the same Canadian team from London, Ontario that our business associate's wife was a member of over 20 years ago. She knew the woman who is now on the board of directors of that team. After trading pins she returned with several of her teammates to introduce me and even invited me to Canada next summer for a dragon boat festival. The next day we ended up racing against the same team. Even though the event is participatory, we were paying attention to our times and places 21st out of 121 teams. Joining over 4,000 breast cancer survivors on the Arno River in Florence was an amazing experience. Being there reinforced that even though we are alone being taken into surgery or sitting in an examining room waiting for test results, we are not alone. When my team had just finished a race and we were getting off the boat, I saw another team headed to the dock. A woman on the team was being carried out of her wheelchair into the boat. Cancer treatment caused her to be too weak to walk. The amazing determination of this paddler made me realize how fortunate we all were to be in Florence being able to physically compete in a sport we were passionate about.

Tips for Trying Dragon Boating

1. Find out if there is a team near you. Dragon boating can be enjoyed by anyone, and there are co-ed teams for everyone as well as teams just for breast cancer survivors and supporters (http://ibcpc.com/).

2. Everyone has had a first time trying dragon boating. Almost everyone involved in the sport is welcoming and friendly. Most teams practice early in the morning on the weekend or in the evening. Sometimes waking up at six a.m. on a Saturday doesn't seem fun. Once I'm on the boat with my

teammates watching the sunrise over the water, it's worth it.

3. Be patient with yourself. Let the team captain know if you have any physical limitations such as needing to avoid paddling on the side you had surgery.

Chapter 10

At Least You Aren't Dead

These words were actually spoken to me. Being dead would be worse. That's true for my own cancer. I'm grateful to still be here. However, others aren't so lucky. Losing loved ones to cancer is awful.

My parents were snowbirds, spending their winters in Florida and summers in Connecticut. Last December I was wondering why my parents were still in snowy New England rather than at their new home in sunny Florida. My mother reported some stomach aches and said she was having tests done. This was not unusual since my mother had a series of health issues over the years such as a blocked carotid artery, stroke, ulcers, migraines, and back issues. In January my parents were still in Connecticut. I was out with my girlfriends when my mother called. It was a Friday night, which was an unusual time for her to call. I stepped outside and said hello. My mother asked if my husband was around. I responded that he was home with the boys and wondered what was happening. She told me she would call back later and I asked for her to let me know what was going on. My mother finally said she needed surgery that was already scheduled. I asked what the surgery was for and she responded, "For the cancer but it will be fine." Excuse me? Did she just say CANCER? My mother had health issues but cancer was never one of them. I asked her if I heard her correctly. Yes, she confirmed. She had stage IV pancreatic cancer.

What!?!?

I proceeded to ask her how long this had been going on. Well, in a roundabout way she told me that she actually knew in December. It seemed like she didn't want to tell me, so our Christmas ski trip wasn't ruined. In typical Jewish mother fashion ("don't worry about me") my mother was dealing with a terminal cancer diagnosis.

Immediately I called my brother in New York City. We planned a trip to Connecticut together to discuss the treatment plan. By the time we arrived, my mother's surgery was canceled. The doctors decided it was too late. Chemo was scheduled. Sitting at the kitchen table in our childhood home, it was evident our mother was dying. Her already pale skin was even paler. She had lost a lot of weight. She was barely eating and had no energy. My mother had been a successful entrepreneur for the past 40 years with a strong personality and New York City sensibility. Seeing her frail and exhausted was difficult.

My brother and I strongly advised my mother not to have chemo. We quickly realized how sick she would be on chemo and how we wouldn't be able to help while living in different states. Our father was clearly overwhelmed, so my brother and I came up with a plan. The chemotherapy scheduled in Hartford would be canceled. My parents would immediately fly to Florida where my mother could enjoy her grandsons, the sunshine, and a few last months without the awful effects of chemotherapy. Thankfully my parents agreed. I called hospice and we picked my parents up at the Palm Beach International Airport with a wheelchair waiting. My mother asked me for water and popped a pain pill. Over the next three months I witnessed the effects of one of the worst types of cancer. Pancreatic cancer causes extreme physical pain. My father coped as best he could seeing his wife of 50 years dying in front of his eyes. Not to mention having different nurses in the house 24/7, having to inject his wife with morphine, and watching her suffer was awful. We placed a hospital bed in the house along with an oxygen tank, walker, and wheelchair.

At one point my mother asked me to make it stop. Although she was slightly delusional on extreme doses of morphine, I understood what she was saying. The pain was unbearable. One night she was screaming in pain. My father and nurses decided to call the ambulance so she could be given a stronger dose of morphine at a local hospice facility. I visited almost everyday, juggling the 35-minute drive with a full time job and two active sons. My brother flew down to visit and she was released after a week. One month later my mother was back in the facility. The end was near. Visiting her was upsetting. We tried talking to her and even turned on her favorite channel, HGTV. Her best friend found a poem she had written for my mom for her 50th birthday. She sent me the poem and asked me to read it to my mom. As my mom lay in bed barely awake I read her friend's sentimental words fighting back the tears. I'm pretty sure she was listening.

One Saturday I was at my son's lacrosse game nearby when the call came.

She was gone.

I was relieved she wasn't in pain anymore, but devastated to lose my 73-year-old mother. My son and I went to the hospice facility to meet my father. I also called my mother-in-law who lived nearby, who I was very close with. Over my many years living in South Florida, she had become like a mother to me. She met me there as well. My son was 11 at the time and he handled it well. We all knew this day would come. After that day I had to quickly make funeral arrangements in Connecticut. Nothing had been pre-planned.

Meanwhile, during this time my mother-in-law was already battling stage IV lung cancer. She had been diagnosed and undergone surgery and chemo for the past four years. However, she looked great and never complained. She even drove herself to chemo, then proceeded to walk around the mall afterwards. She was also very active raising money as president of her local Pap Corps chapter. Named for famed physician Dr. Papanicolaou, who invented the Pap smear, the organization raises funds for Sylvester Comprehensive Cancer Center at the University of Miami Medical School.

This past Thanksgiving we went on a family cruise with four of my mother-in-law's grandchildren and even my widowed father. When a cruise begins, they perform a "muster" drill. All passengers must line up on the deck of the ship for about 20 minutes. After five minutes, my mother-in-law could no longer stand. She collapsed to the ship floor and we took her inside. She was very weak but still enjoyed the cruise. Her and her husband of over 60 years managed to dance one last time to a live mambo band in front of their family. When we returned, her health deteriorated quickly. The cancer was spreading. Once again hospice was called. My mother-in-law was given morphine. One day I went to visit and the memory of my mother less than a year before hit me. This was a repeat of what just occurred with my own mother. The morphine, the hospice nurses, the oxygen tanks. I couldn't believe it. I suddenly felt an enormous sense of anger and sorrow. How could this be happening again? My mother in law died this spring just before her 81st birthday. Both mothers are missed everyday.

Although they are gone, knowing that they are no longer in pain is a relief.

How can my sons lose both grandmothers to cancer within a year? My husband and I both were fortunate to have our grandmothers attend our wedding. Mine lived until 92 years old and his passed away at 101. It is sad that my sons will not experience a longer relationship with their grandmothers. One of the lessons learned from these amazing women is to live life to the fullest. Whether it is called carpe diem or "YOLO" (you only live once), it is important to remember that we all are only here for a short time. Cancer has taught me to enjoy life. After all, at least I'm not dead.

Tips for Dealing with Loss

1. Respect the wishes of the person who is suffering. My mother requested that her clothes be donated to Dress for Success. It took me a long time to sort through the closets in both of her houses. Finally, when I dropped off outfits to the organization that helps underprivileged women prepare for job interviews, I knew my mom would have been pleased.

2. Take time for yourself to process and think about what is happening. Connect with your spiritual self.

3. Plan ahead—take care of details such as funeral arrangements, obituaries, eulogies, etc. beforehand if possible.

Chapter 11

How to Speak with Children

Be honest with kids. They want to know the truth. Being open with children is helpful. They want to know in simple terms: are you going to die? How does the cancer affect them? How will their lives change? The first time I had cancer, my children weren't born yet. The second time around, they were nine and ten. They knew what cancer was and that I already had cancer. We had attended funerals of relatives who had died of cancer. I was honest with them, assuring them I would be fine but needed surgery. During the mastectomy my parents took care of the boys in New York City and they came to visit me in the hospital. When I was home recovering from all of my surgeries, the boys were supportive. Friends, family, and neighbors provided a helping hand. As I recovered I was searching for cancer resources on the Internet and stumbled across Camp Kesem. The website said that it was a non-profit organization supporting kids who have a parent going through cancer where "kids can be kids."

Founded by college students at Stanford University in 2000, they recognized that over five million children in the U.S. are impacted by a parent's cancer diagnosis. A one-week free summer sleepaway camp experience was created to support the needs of this overlooked population. Led entirely by college students, Camp Kesem has expanded to over 105 chapters in 40 states. I applied to our closest chapter at the University of Miami. The program rents out a traditional summer camp on a lake in central Florida. This year our sons attended their fourth year of Camp Kesem. It is truly their favorite part of the summer. Both boys have decided they will be Kesem counselors when they are older. When we attend reunions during the year, the dedication that these college student have for Camp Kesem is amazing. The students even offer to attend kids' birthday parties and sports activities during the year. We feel truly fortunate to have discovered and become a part of this community.

Tips For Discussing Cancer With Children

1. Be honest. It is worse for children to guess what is wrong with their loved one. One of my teachers told me that my son said I had the flu when I was actually diagnosed with breast cancer. I couldn't believe it. Why would he think that? Since I wasn't

sure how to explain it, I just said that mommy was sick and was very aloof. Breast cancer isn't easy to explain to a ten-year-old boy. When I sat him down and explained what was happening, he seemed to be relieved even though I was going in for surgery.

2. Let them express their feelings. Acknowledge their emotions whether they are sad, scared, or angry. During my mother's funeral, one of my sons stood in the corner of the funeral home reception room in his three-piece suit bawling. My other son did not cry and was chatting with relatives. Each child expresses emotions differently and that's OK.

3. Allow kids to be kids—Camp Kesem is an amazing break for kids who have parents or grandparents going through cancer. The time for children to unplug, have fun, and be themselves around other kids and away from their parents is important. My sons always return from Camp Kesem a bit more considerate and kind. If there is not a Kesem chapter near you, think about what opportunities you can provide your children to enjoy life without the stress and sadness of cancer, even if just for a little while. http://campkesem.org/

Chapter 12

How to Live

What does a healthy life mean to you? I thought I was healthy when I was diagnosed with thyroid cancer at the age of 29. A recent article posted on social media cited some of the causes of cancer: smoking, drinking alcohol, eating too much red meat and being overweight. Reading these articles are frustrating to me. I have never smoked (maybe I tried it a few times,) I'm not a big drinker, I've never been overweight and I was a vegetarian in high school. Since being diagnosed I have exercised, eaten more nutritiously, and had two children. My thyroid was checked every six months and I thought I was healthy. Then in 2015 I was diagnosed with breast cancer at the age of 42. Like most women I was busy with my family, work, friends, and life. I didn't have time for cancer again. Now I'm recovering from my sixth cancer-related surgery. There are days I don't feel like exercising. Staying in bed is tempting. Popsicles are more comforting than carrots. What's a cancer survivor to do?

The following tips are some things that worked for me. For convenience, I've separated them into six sections:

1. Nutrition
2. Healthcare
3. Physical Activity
4. Staying Positive
5. Inner Peace
6. Stress Relief

Nutrition

Meet with a Nutritionist or Health Coach

If you would like to improve your eating habits, a nutritionist or health coach can help to guide you. Fortunately my sister-in-law in New York City is a nutritionist and always has advice on everything from healthy snacks to organic delivery services. There is also a plethora of free nutrition advice on the Internet such as cancer-fighting foods and recipes. Turmeric is an Indian spice that acts as an anti-inflammatory and antioxidant and even fights cancer. This can easily be added to daily cooking like sauteed vegetables or even your morning eggs. If the taste doesn't appeal to you, supplements are also available. When recovering from surgery be sure to eat enough protein even if you aren't hungry. My brother brought me bone broth which is rich in minerals and protein, fights inflammation, and helps digestion. Bone broth is sold at most health food stores and your local green market.

Eat Organic

Eat organic when possible, especially for the "Dirty Dozen." These are fruits and vegetables that contain the most pesticides. Since being diagnosed I am more aware of eating organic and even make sure that my morning coffee is organic, since coffee beans are one of the most chemically treated foods in the world. Exposure to large amounts of pesticides have been linked to many types of cancer. I wash all of my produce with an organic vegie spray.

Limit Sugar and White Flours

Many studies have concluded that sugar feeds cancer. Do not eat sugary foods and use natural replacements for sugar such as Stevia. My acupuncturist gave me some sage advice: increase protein intake, limit eating carbs at night, and hot foods are healthier than cold. Although I'm not a dessert fan, I love carbs and could live on bread. In fact, I did live on fresh bread and pasta when I was living in Belgium in graduate school. These days my diet has changed to include protein in the morning, even if it is in a smoothie or eating an egg bite on the way to the office. I also try to avoid gluten, white flour, and sugar.

<u>Do What Works for You</u>

There are so many diets available for cancer, health, weight loss, and longevity. Sometimes the amount of information can be overwhelming. The ketogenic diet, grapefruit diet, low carb, high protein, and vegan diets can all be useful to some people. Eating should be more of a lifestyle than a short-term diet.

<u>Make Your Own Food</u>

Although the convenience of buying prepared food is hard to resist, making your own can be healthier and less expensive. My husband bought me a juicer which was fun at first. However it takes almost an entire pound of carrots to make a glass of juice. The cleanup is time consuming. If you want to buy a juicer, be sure to get one that doesn't remove the healthful fiber. Eating whole fruits and veggies is always the best choice.

When I didn't have an appetite, smoothies were a great way to be nourished. A good blender can make any type of smoothie. Begin with an organic protein powder, add water or a nut milk, ice, a banana, and your favorite frozen fruit. You can even add kale, apples, green powder, collagen powder, etc. The list is endless. If you are taking Synthroid, be sure not to have any soy products within four hours after taking it since it interferes with the drug's absorption. I avoid all soy products since there have been some studies linking soy to higher estrogen levels in breast cancer patients. Soy contains isoflavones which are plant estrogens. The studies are mixed about this. One of my doctors said, "Go ahead and have your soy latte once in a while." I prefer not to take the chance. Instead of ice cream, I blend a frozen banana with almond or peanut butter which is surprisingly rich and satisfying.

Healthcare

Keep Records

Maintain proper record keeping of all surgeries, medication, diagnosis, etc. It is extremely helpful to have a system to store your records. Lab results, doctor's reports, images, and insurance documents should all be saved in one place and easily accessible. My father is very fastidious, keeping records of everything from when he took his vitamins, his weekly weight and blood test results all in a notebook. Either use a binder with all papers in chronological order or electronically scan or photograph all documents and place in a cloud service such as Dropbox, OneNote, or Evernote. There are also apps that will keep track of your records. Each time I went to a new doctor, I had to complete several pages of medical history. Having multiple surgeries, it can be difficult to remember dates. Keeping the information readily available makes everything quicker and easier. One time when the nurse handed me a clipboard with a five-page questionnaire of medical history, I handed the blank paper back with a pre-printed page of all of my surgeries, diagnoses, and current medication. It was clear that they weren't used to being given something like that from a patient.

You're in Charge

Get a second and third opinion: be your own advocate. Ask questions and seek referrals from other patients. Bring a friend or relative with you to appointments for support.

Understand Insurance

Dealing with insurance companies can be a full-time job. Once diagnosed, ask your insurance company about your benefits. If you are seeking care out of state, verify the percentage insurance will cover. Also keep in mind that the medical bills are separate for the hospital, doctor's office, anesthesiologist, etc. I have learned that hospital bills can be paid off in increments without interest penalties. For example, if the hospital asks for payment the day of your surgery, ask if you can pay half now and half at a later date. Almost every hospital I asked has agreed to this without a penalty. Some employers are now offering cancer insurance policies. Check to see if there is a clause for a pre existing condition. For patients without health insurance, there are government funded hospitals, Medicare and Medicaid, and non profit organizations that can assist with cancer-related costs. Getting into credit card debt to handle health care costs is adding undue stress to an already stressful situation. A non profit organization called Nancy's List launched by a patient provides comprehensive information for financial resources: https://nancyslist.org/financial-assistance/.

Find a Doctor You Trust

Looking back, finding a capable and qualified physician was really challenging. My advice is to ask friends and family, contact your state's cancer hospitals, or contact local support groups for recommendations and information.

Seek Alternative Medicine Options

Combining traditional medicine with alternative treatments is extremely common. As long as the alternative treatments weren't harmful, I was willing to try just about everything from acupuncture to drinking tea made of dead bugs. At one point I was taking over 40 supplements per day. Colonics were recommended to me so I tried that as well. Today I only take a few regular supplements and continue with acupuncture when needed (I canceled a surgery to repair my torn meniscus when acupuncture healed my knee). My oncologist is currently giving me B12 injections every month, which gives me more energy. Figure out what holistic medicine works for you in combination with traditional medicine.

Physical Activity

Walking and Running

Even if your doctor instructs you to limit vigorous exercise, walking is usually acceptable. Although limiting my activity is really challenging, staying active is important. I remember forcing myself to walk around the block when recovering from surgery and always felt better afterwards. If it is too hot or raining, I go on the treadmill.

Yoga

The power of yoga is really amazing. The practice can range from extremely flexible yogis doing headstands and sweating in a heated studio to gentle breathing and slow movements (more of my pace). My husband's grandmother was doing headstands in the 1970s when yoga wasn't well-known. She was also a dancer, a vegetarian and lived until 101 years old.

Sedentary Modalities

Sitting is the new smoking. Americans sit more than most other cultures. Recent studies have proven that it isn't how much we sit, but rather the way we sit, that is the problem. This causes back problems and can lead to spinal disc issues. Both of my parents suffered from back problems for years. They even had ruptured discs and required surgery. Yoga, pilates, and a good chiropractor can help with these issues. Strengthening your core can also help. I have a friend who is a professional equestrian rider, and her posture is the best I've ever seen. Also, sitting on an exercise ball instead of a chair, taking walking breaks, or even getting a standing desk, can help improve posture. Although back pain has nothing to do with cancer, overall health is important.

Staying Positive

Self-Help Books and Seminars

As a college student, my mother introduced me to my first motivational seminar. Stephen Covey wrote a book called *Seven Habits of Highly Effective People*. He was a dynamic speaker and this led to my interest in the self-help genre. Five years ago, my mom sent me to a five-day Jack Canfield seminar called *Breakthrough to Success* in Arizona. After getting through cancer I wanted to learn how to live my best life. This experience led me to offer retreats for women and become a cancer coach. After all, the past and future are not actually happening. All we have is the present moment.

<u>Support Groups</u>

Join a support group. Not everyone is comfortable sharing their medical history with a room full of strangers. The comfort of knowing that others are facing similar issues can be beneficial. They can also help provide answers to questions about surgery or treatment. Every cancer patient worries about recurrence, whether they were diagnosed one year ago or ten years ago. Each time we go for a test, it is natural to think about the worst case scenario. As my husband often says, "Worry is a misuse of the imagination." Rather than thinking about a recurrence, try to imagine the doctor telling you about being cancer-free and plan for a celebration.

<u>Avoid Negativity</u>

Stay away from negative people. After fighting a serious disease, you may realize how important it is to surround yourself with positive people. Anyone who is negative or emotionally draining is not worth your time. Nurture relationships with family and friends who are supportive and do the same for them. Several studies (including a well-known Harvard study featured in a TED Talk) have proven that one of the keys to a happy life is quality relationships. (https://ideas.ted.com/4-lessons-from-the-longest-running-study-on-happiness/)

Inner Peace

Meditation

Meditation can be an integral part of healing. When I received radiation I imagined the cancer cells being "eaten" by Pacman-looking creatures. Each morning I use an app called Calm. This is a paid app that provides a new ten-minute morning meditation every single day. The app also tracks your meditation progress and provides bedtime stories if you have trouble sleeping. There are also many free meditation videos on YouTube.

Reiki

Reiki is a Japanese energy healing technique promoting emotional and physical healing. My friend in Colorado is a licensed reiki master and performed it on me. She told me that she sensed a waterfall sensation during the session when I was lying still. Sure enough, I hadn't mentioned that my breast implant had contracted due to the high altitude causing an alarming sloshing sound when I moved it. A free program for a similar modality called Healing Touch was offered locally to cancer patients so I tried it. I found it to be very relaxing and believe it's worth your time.

Survivor-Focused Classes

When I was in too much pain to attend my regular yoga class, I searched for classes tailored to cancer survivors. Initially, I wasn't sure if they even existed. But I ended up finding one! A local studio offered a donation-based class twice a week for cancer patients. If you can't do a pose, the instructor offers alternatives. This class has been a big part of my healing process. If you aren't ready to go to a studio, stretching out at home can do wonders for the body and mind. When I was doing physical therapy at a local hospital after the mastectomy, they offered chair yoga. It was a free class and since I wasn't allowed to practice a strenuous yoga class yet, I decided to go. Although the average participant age was 80, we spent an hour exercising, all while sitting in a chair!

Stress Relief

Delegate

I'll admit that I think I can "do it all," then suffer from stress when it isn't possible. My Virgo personality strives for perfection which is not always a good trait. Learning how to give out tasks to family members, friends, or hired help is important. Especially when a patient is healing, asking for help is critical. Don't be afraid to ask neighbors for help if your children need rides or for a friend to bring food when you are too tired to cook. When a friend dropped off my favorite homemade Indian dinner once when I was recovering, it was really meaningful and helpful. An organization called Cleaning for a

Reason provides free house cleaning when you are too tired from cancer to do it yourself or your medical bills prevent you from hiring someone. Simple things like walking the dog isn't possible when recovering from a mastectomy. If the dog pulls you on the leash you could risk damage. When a friend or relative is facing cancer and you are not sure how to react or what to do, the best thing is to provide unsolicited help. Most people have difficulty asking for help. Offer to bring a meal, walk their dog, or give their child a ride. My closest friend stayed with me after reconstructive surgery. She made my meals and we spent most of the time lounging on the couch and chatting. This was invaluable to my recovery.

Spend Time in Nature

Nature provides a free and therapeutic type of stress relief. Whether you live near mountains, lakes, rivers, or the ocean, go for a walk. Just a simple walk in the woods or even around the block can lift spirits. Leave your cell phone at home and listen to the birds or the sound of the waves. This sounds so easy, however too many people go from their house to their workplace and back to the house again. I live ten minutes from the beach and there are times when weeks pass without seeing the ocean. At Memorial Sloan Kettering and many other cancer hospitals, nature scene channels are available on the televisions. Hearing the sound of a river flowing over rocks is more soothing than watching the news. Sometimes we need to force ourselves to take the time to enjoy the natural world around us. Not only is it enjoyable, it can also be healing.

Pet Therapy

Pets are proven to reduce stress. Just petting a dog can calm us down. When my mother was in hospice, a physician brought her therapy dogs to the facility. My father still talks about how nice those dogs were. Seeing furry friends can really lift spirits in an otherwise dark time. My colleague at the college where I teach brings his service dog to the office. It doesn't matter if you are having a bad or good day, this fluffy golden retriever greets everyone and always seems to have a smile on his face. The students enjoy having him in class. Being in a bad mood is difficult when you see a cute dog who just wants some attention. My little poodle has always been by my side when I'm in bed recovering from one of my surgeries. She loves to lay right beside me and put her head on the pillow.

Even if you don't have a pet, local shelters are always seeking volunteers to walk dogs or even play with the cats. These animals don't care if you have scars or are tired, they provide unconditional love. A new trend has swept the country demonstrating the healing power of animals. Goat yoga is an actual class offered in barns, parks, and even urban yoga studios. Combining adorable baby goats who climb all over the participants while in downward dog is the perfect combination to uplift one's spirits. Although I babysat goats in high school and didn't enjoy them butting me while I was trying to feed them, the class sounds intriguing.

Limit Screen Time

I ask my college students how many of them have their cell phones next to them when they are sleeping. Usually about 90 percent raise their hands. Since cell phones also double as alarm clocks and radios, we keep them close. However, the blue light emitted can stimulate the brain and curb our ability to sleep. Sometimes the urge to check your email one last time or even the social media feed is tempting. Try to limit screen time before bed. If you think screen time is taking away from family time this can also create stress. Easy to implement rules can be helpful. Growing up, my mother would take the phone "off the hook" during dinner. Along the same theme, I don't allow cell phones or iPads when we are eating at home or in a restaurant. Some of our most fun family memories is surprisingly during hurricanes. Living in South Florida we experience serious tropical storms and hurricanes every few years. Without cable, WiFi, and sometimes power, kids and neighbors get together, play board games, and have fun without the distraction of electronics.

<u>Medical Marijuana and CBD Oil</u>
Medical marijuana is currently legal in 30 states. Some studies suggest that marijuana can actually kill cancer cells. It can also help with the side effects of chemotherapy, anxiety, sleeping, and pain. CBD (cannabidiol) is an oil derived from cannabis that has benefits without the side effect of feeling "stoned" because of the absence of THC. For every one of my surgeries I was prescribed either Oxycodone or Vicodin. Both drugs are very powerful and make me nauseated and uncomfortable. Many patients are experiencing better results with cannabis. Do your research to be sure what you are using is pure. The CBD oil business has grown exponentially in recent years. Whether you are trying medical marijuana or CBD oil, be sure that it is legal and safe.

Even More Tips for Moving Forward

1. Take a walk. Even when I don't feel well, I force myself to walk around the block or on the beach using my headphones with uplifting music. This is guaranteed to help me feel better.

2. Join a cause. After my diagnosis I looked for something to prove to myself that cancer couldn't

stop me. I joined a dragon boating team of breast cancer survivors. Paddling a boat in unison with other women who went through breast cancer is empowering! After practice we compare notes on surgery, doctors, and experiences.

3. Take a breath. Meditation is very powerful. Going into surgery at Sloan Kettering, I listened to a meditation for surgery recording on my headphones. This helped me to be calm and at peace. There are free meditation apps available for download to help you with everything from sleep to life balance.

In Closing

The Journey

A friend recently asked if I was angry.

Why should I be angry?

She responded that I have had cancer twice and six surgeries.

No, I'm not angry. I'm actually thankful.

Of course, I am angry at losing both of my mothers to cancer. I am angry that my good friend's 15-year-old son has bone cancer. I am angry that a woman I played tennis with for the past several years just died of breast cancer. I am angry that a cure for cancer doesn't seem to be happening.

But, I'm still here and am more motivated than ever to make a difference. I'm a national speaker, author, cancer coach, and patient advocate. Without cancer, I wouldn't have discovered dragon boating or made any friends without the commonality of cancer. My sons are more empathetic after seeing their mother and grandmothers endure cancer. Camp Kesem has become an important aspect in my children's lives.

I still go to the oncologist once a month for B12 injections. These provide energy and help to strengthen the immune system. Looking around the waiting room is a harsh reminder of cancer. There are patients who lost their hair, patients in wheelchairs, and patients of different colors and ages. My injections are given in the chemo room, which really puts everything into perspective. Watching other patients settle into the oversized chairs for hours of treatment, I watch the nurses prepare tubes and needles. Never having chemo myself, I wonder how they endure it. Then I realize that being worried about rushing off to where I am going after my appointment (usually work or picking up my kids) isn't worth stressing over. I should be thankful. Cancer is more that just an annoying part of my day.

Cancer hasn't defined me.

If you are recently diagnosed, a survivor, or a supporter, I encourage you to not allow cancer to define you. Participate in activities you enjoy if you are able. A seminar I once attended handed out two envelopes: one labeled "worries" and one labeled "grateful." The audience was asked to list as many things as they were worried about in five minutes. Then, everything they were grateful for went into the second envelope. This process actually helps you to forget your worries and realize the blessings in your life. Many meditations suggest that we think about one thing we are grateful for before getting out of bed each day. For example, if you are tired and don't want to go to work, change the conversation. I think: "I'm grateful to work with wonderful colleagues and to influence the lives of students."

Cancer is just part of my journey.

Warren Buffett, the billionaire investor, has an insightful outlook on taking care of ourselves. In the 2017 HBO documentary *Becoming Warren Buffett,* the 80-year old said, "What car would you like to have if I offered you any car? The catch: It is the only car you are going to get in your lifetime. Since it is your only car, you are going to have to take care of it. We should think about our body and minds the same as this vehicle. We only get one mind and body, and they may feel terrific now, but it must last you a lifetime. Make sure you are thinking long-term with the decisions that affect your body and mind."

We have a responsibility to take care of our health for our family, friends, and ultimately ourselves. My aunt in Albuquerque is in her 80s with no major health issues. She was a successful business woman before entrepreneurship was trendy. Since her husband passed away she lives alone, has a boyfriend and a zest for life. I recently asked her what her secret is. The response: "My Jane Fonda workout every day, a daily multivitamin, and plenty of sex." Amazing. One of my favorite quotes about health is from the Dalai Lama, who I was privileged to hear speak at my nephew's graduation from Tulane University. In reference to when asked what surprised him about humanity, he responded, "Man. Because he sacrifices his health in order to make money. Then he sacrifices his money to recuperate his health. And then he is so anxious about the future that he does not enjoy the present; the result being that he does not live in the present or future; he lives as if he is never going to die, then dies having never really lived." Be sure to put your health first. Be your own advocate. Create meaningful relationships. Enjoy activities you are passionate about. We only have one life. After my dragon boat race in Florence this summer, we drove to Genoa, Italy on our way to Monaco and France. A few weeks later the same bridge we drove on collapsed, killing 38 people. My husband and I discussed this and decided it just wasn't our time.

During both cancer experiences some friends stopped communicating. I think they were not sure what to do or say. I certainly don't blame those friends for staying away from a scary situation. If you have a friend or relative dealing with cancer, a simple call or text to let them know you are thinking about them can go a long way. Offer to talk or get together if they are up to it. Sometimes that's all a patient needs.

Perhaps one day cancer will be cured.

But until then, live your life to the fullest.

To me cancer isn't a fight.

There are no winners.

My intention is to face cancer with strength and gratitude.

About Marla

Marla Friedman is a best-selling author, national speaker, and cancer coach. She is dedicated to helping patients, survivors, and their families through cancer. Marla founded ThyCa South Florida in 2001—a chapter of the Thyroid Cancer Survivor's Association. She continues to support newly diagnosed patients and speak at national conferences. She also volunteers with the Sharsheret Organization, supporting young Jewish women with breast and ovarian cancer. In 2014 Marla launched Weekend Getaways for Women, a retreat company for busy women offering seminars on relationships, vision boards, yoga and makeovers. Marla is a founding member of Lighthouse Dragons SOS dragon boat team in Jupiter, FL. The team is comprised of breast cancer survivors and supporters. Marla and her team competed in Florence, Italy in the International Dragon Boat Festival in July of 2018 with 4,000 other breast cancer survivors from all over the world. Dr. Friedman is a full-time business and entrepreneurship professor at Palm Beach State College. She is a also a consultant advising business owners how to create their strategic competitive advantage. She also contributed a story to

Conversations That Make a Difference: Stories that Support a Bigger Vision, a 2014 Amazon best seller. This compilation project included Marla's story of growing up with a mother who valued entrepreneurship.

Marla earned a bachelor's degree in public relations and a master's degree in global marketing communications & advertising; both from Emerson College. Her doctoral degree is in higher education education leadership from Nova Southeastern University. Marla resides in Palm Beach Gardens, FL with her husband, two sons and miniature poodle.

If you'd like to learn more about Marla, feel free to visit her website, www.thegoodcancer.com or contact her via email: drmarlaf@gmail.com.

Thank You From Story Ninjas

Story Ninjas Publishing would like to thank you for reading this book. We hope you found value in our product and would love to hear your feedback. We would love to hear your constructive criticism in a review on Amazon. Also feel free to share this book with your friends and family through the various social media platforms.

Other Books by Story Ninjas

Story Ninjas Publishing hopes you enjoyed this book. Check out our Amazon page for more products you may be interested in.

About Story Ninjas

Story Ninjas Publishing is an independent book publisher. Our stories range from science fiction to paranormal romance. Our goal is to create stories that are not only entertaining, but endearing. We believe engaging narrative can lead to personal growth. Through unforgettable characters and powerful plot we portray themes that are relevant for today's issues.

You can find more Story Ninja's products here.

Follow Story Ninjas!!!
Website: www.story-ninjas.com
Email: Story-Ninjas@Story-Ninjas.com
Twitter: @StoryNinjas
Youtube: @StoryNinjas
Amazon: Story Ninjas
G+: +Story Ninjas
Facebook: StoryNinjasHQ
LinkedIn: Story-Ninjas
Blogger: Story-NinjasHQ

SELECTED BIBLIOGRAPHY

Beckett, S. (1954). Waiting for Godot. 1954. Samuel Beckett: The Complete Dramatic Works, 7-89.

Byrne, R. (2008). The secret. Simon and Schuster.

Goodrich, F., & Hackett, A. (1958). The Diary of Anne Frank. Dramatists Play Service, Inc..

Hay, L. L. (2009). You can heal your life. ReadHowYouWant. Com.

Kunhardt, P. Oakes, B. Kunhardt, T. Kunhardt, G. (2017). *Becoming Warren Buffett* [Video]. https://www.amazon.com/Becoming-Warren-Buffett/dp/B01MSBOHUM

Phillips, C. (2010). Socrates Cafe: A Fresh Taste of Philosophy: A Fresh Taste of Philosophy. WW Norton & Company.

Redfield, J. (2013). The celestine prophecy. Random
House.

Wiesel, E., & Wiesel, M. (2008). The night trilogy:
Night ; Dawn ; Day / Elie Wiesel. New York:
Hill and Wang.

Made in the USA
Middletown, DE
27 May 2019